OBESITY

Worldwide

I0113551

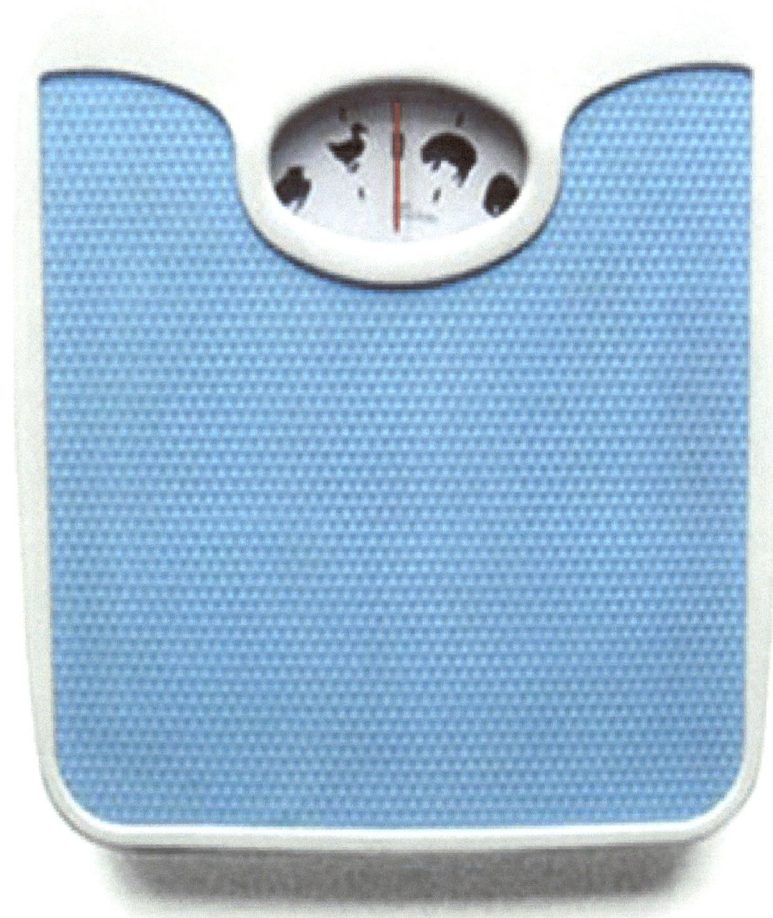

By: Oliver Greene

Published by New Generation Publishing in 2013

Copyright © Oliver Greene 2013

First Edition

The author asserts the moral right under the Copyright, Designs and Patents Act 1988 to be identified as the author of this work.

All Rights reserved. No part of this publication may be reproduced, stored in a retrieval system or transmitted, in any form or by any means without the prior consent of the author, nor be otherwise circulated in any form of binding or cover other than that which it is published and without a similar condition being imposed on the subsequent purchaser.

www.newgeneration-publishing.com

New Generation Publishing

By: Oliver Greene

Contents

By: Oliver Greene

Introduction

Unpredictably, it is our survival skills that are killing us. Our eating habits and lifestyle are turning our bodies into fat-hoarding machines. Food was indeed for survival for our ancestors, especially when they were unsure about what their next meal would be. But with access to jam-packed junk food aisles and drive-through restaurants, the mechanism of survival is wreaking havoc on our health.

Obesity is a complicated and multi-factorial disease that is basically developed through the interaction between the environment and genotype. Obesity is recognized as both a lifestyle disorder and a medical condition falling within the context of family, individual and societal functioning. While the understanding of obesity occurrence is still incomplete, it is believed to involve the integration of behavioral, social, metabolic, physiological, cultural, and genetic factors.

Fortunately, today healthcare practitioners are taking the responsibility to provide better obesity management. In fact, many physicians are encouraged to seek guidance for providing effective treatment methods to fight the growing obesity epidemic.

Treatment of an obese or overweight person incorporates a two-step procedure: management and assessment. Management not only involves maintenance of body weight and weight loss, but it also incorporates preventative measures from risk factors. On the other hand, assessment involves the determination of obesity and its overall impact on the health status.

By: Oliver Greene

Obesity is growing at an alarming rate. It is affecting not only a few countries but our planet as a whole. Moreover, the velocity of its rise will not stop increasing until we change our sedentary lifestyle and our bad eating habits. No one can help us more than ourselves. Every day, we can make choices to eat and move for a longer and healthier life.

An entire generation is growing up in an obesogenic environment in which the forces behind sedentary behavior are growing, not declining.

This book is an attempt to educate people to bring a decline in the growing epidemic of obesity to create a un-obesogenic environment for our upcoming generation, so it can live a healthier and longer life.

By: Oliver Greene

The Alarming Obesity Situation

Obesity is "an excess of body fat frequently resulting in a significant impairment of health and longevity", according to the Faculty of Public Health. The common way to assess body fat is by 'body mass index' (BMI) which is calculated by dividing an individual's weight measured in kilograms by their height in meters squared. The following is the BMI chart that classifies Body Mass Index in detail.

Classification	BMI (kg/m^2)
Underweight	<18.5
Normal Range	18.5 – 24.9
Overweight	25.0 – 29.0
Obese	>30.0
Obese Class I	30.0 – 34.9
Obese Class II	35.0 – 39.9
Obese Class III	>40.0

BMI is considered a reliable indicator of body fat. Although it does not measure the direct body fat, but according to research the BMI correlates to direct body fat measurements. In addition, BMI is an easy-to-perform and inexpensive way for screening weight and its consequences to health condition.

BMI is basically used as a screening tool to recognize the possible overweight problems for adult and children. However, it should not be used as a diagnostic

By: Oliver Greene

tool. For example, all overweight or obese people may not have similar health consequences.

In order to determine the particular health problem one is suffering due to excessive weight, a proper health diagnosis must take place. The assessments usually include family history, physical activity, evaluation of diet, skin-fold thickness measurements, and other appropriate health screenings.

How reliable is BMI as a Body Fat Indicator?

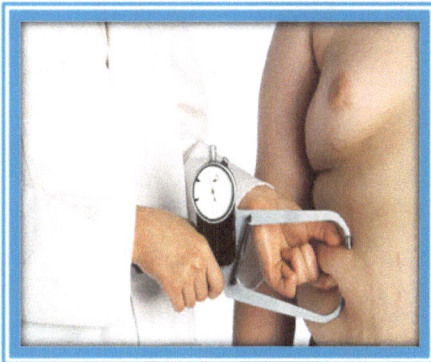

The correlation between the body fat and BMI is very strong. However, the strength of the correlation varies by age, race, and sex. For example:

- Women tend to have more body fat as compared to men, at the same body mass index level.
- As compared to younger adults, older people tend to have more body fat, at the same BMI.
- Athletes and body builders tend to have higher BMI due to excessive muscularity rather than excessive body fatness.

Also note that BMI is the only factor related to the risk for disease.

The Obesity Problem

Excessive fat in the body or obesity has become one of the biggest problems of this century. Obesity has been divided into three different stages:

- Pitiable
- Laughable
- Enviable

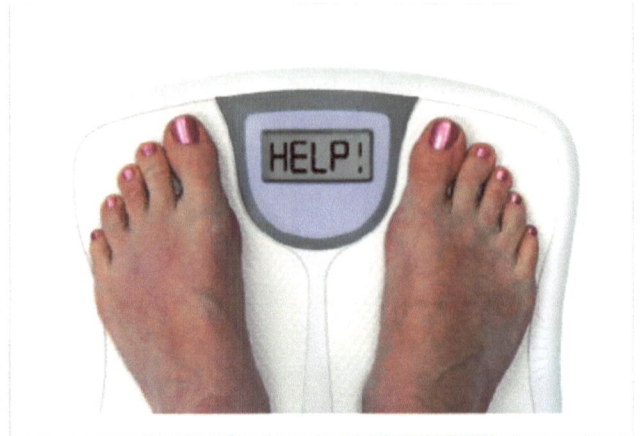

The enviable stage is one in which the little extra weight makes you look more smooth, round and beautiful (although, the concept of beauty changes with time). However, in the next stage, i.e. the laughable stage, people start laughing at your excessive weight which makes you look bulky and ugly. And when this stage moves on to the level of severity where it gets impossible for the person to get up or move around without help, it is the pitiable stage.

There are several reasons why excessive fat accumulation makes you overweight or obese. In some cases, it is the organic cause that is functioning. For example, lack of thyroid hormone or excess of female sex hormone or adrenal cortisone can cause obesity.

While in some cases, obesity is caused due to damage to the lower part of the brain which controls satisfaction and hunger. However, the majority of the cases do not belong to these categories. In the majority of cases, the clear blame of obesity is given to the modern lifestyle.

By: Oliver Greene

But what factors of our modern lifestyle contribute to obesity?

In short, our body is similar to a plastic bag, the size of which is determined by what you put inside and what you take out. For example, the amount of calories you put in and the amount of calories you burn/take out by daily activities and exercise determines the size of your body.

Our modern lifestyle is loaded with advanced technology and busy schedules. In short, our life has become sedentary. Therefore, we are left with no time to engage in any physical activity or physical work. Many of us are into a lot of brainwork, which burns fewer calories than engaging in physical activity such as playing, running, walking, etc.

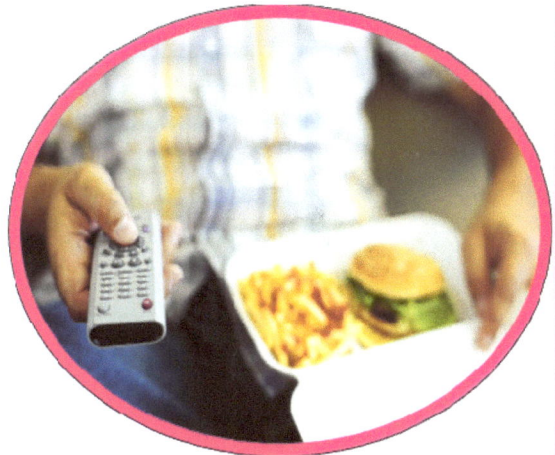

According to scientists, "telling obese people to 'just eat less' is equivalent of advising a chronic heroin addict to 'cut down a bit'. In addition to lazy and sedentary lifestyle, addiction to food is also contributing towards the growing epidemic of obesity worldwide.

Obesity is growing at an alarming rate while many people are still unaware of the reasons and consequences. Only in the United States, 97 million adults are estimated to be either overweight or obese. These conditions eventually increase the substantial risk of morbidity from dyslipidemia, hypertension, type II diabetes, stroke, coronary artery disease, gallbladder disease, sleep apnea, respiratory problem, osteoarthritis, as well as cancers of the colon, prostate, breast, and

By: Oliver Greene

endometrium. Excessive body weight is also associated with an increase in mortality from all causes.

Did You Know?
Obesity is the second leading cause of death, the first being tobacco.

Obese people may also suffer from discrimination and other social stigmatization. Today, excessive weight and obesity has become a major cause of preventable death around the globe. Obesity poses a major public health challenge.

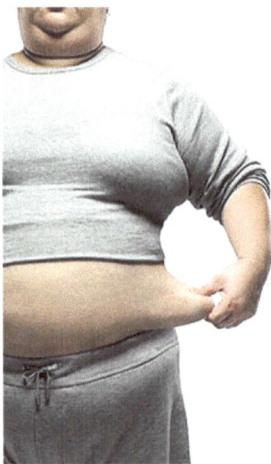

Obesity and overweight cannot be considered mutually exclusive. This is because all obese people are also overweight. If a Body Mass Indicator of 30 means 30 excessive pounds, it can be exemplified in several ways. Either it's about a person who is five feet and six inches tall with weight of 186 pound, or it could be a 6 feet tall person with weight of 186 pounds.

The number of obese and overweight men and women has risen dramatically since 1960. The most evident groups suffering this epidemic are some minority groups and people with less education and lower incomes.

There are several reasons why the presence of obesity or excessive weight in a patient is of medical concern. Such people become susceptible to several diseases, particularly diabetes mellitus and cardiovascular diseases.

Indeed, modern lifestyle is the main reason that obesity is growing so aggressively. The primary culprits of obesity should be controlled in order to control the growing epidemic. People should be aware of 'why it is happening' and 'with whom it is happening' to prevent it.

By: Oliver Greene

Classification and Assessment of Obesity

Although people show agreement when it comes to health risks associated with obesity and excessive weight, the agreement changes to disagreement when it comes to managing these health risks.

People are seen arguing against treating obesity or reducing excessive weight considering the difficulty in achieving weight loss and maintaining it on a long-term basis. Moreover, these people talk about the negative consequences of weight cycling. They argue that the potential hazards of treating obesity do not offset the hazards of being obese.

Such approach is due to lack of information, education, and reluctance. Treatment of obese and overweight patients is basically a two-step procedure – assessment and management.

- **Assessment** – the requirement of absolute risk status and the determination of the degree of obesity.
- **Management** – includes weight reduction and maintaining lower body weight together with controlling related risk factors.

Treating obesity indeed requires time and effort. Obesity is a chronic disease and therefore the patients must understand that it requires a lifelong effort to successfully treat obesity and its related health hazards.

By: Oliver Greene

There are some accurate methods available to determine the exact body fat. However, measuring body fat through these techniques is quite expensive and not readily available. This is why there are two surrogate measures that are commonly used to assess body fat. These are:

- Body Mass Index
- Waist Circumference

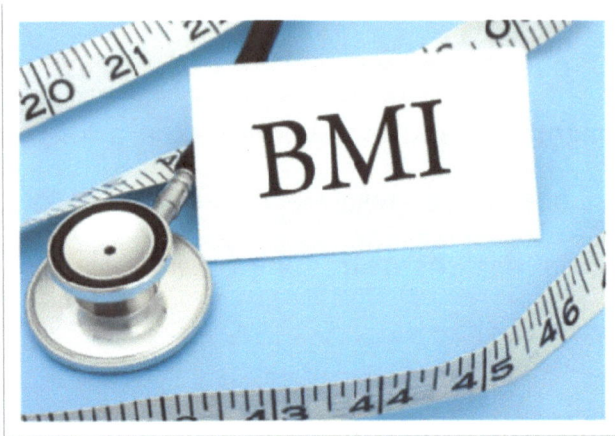

BMI is a very common fat measurement technique. It is a very practical approach considering body fat assessment. BMI provides accurate body fat as compared to the total body weight. However, BMI has certain limitations. For example, the results are based on generic data. It over-estimates body fat for people who are muscular. On the other hand, it under-estimates BMI for people who have lost muscle mass. In a nutshell, BMI does not incorporate all relevant factors about a person and only gives results on the basis of height and weight.

Waist Circumference is another most used practical tool to determine the abdominal fat of a person. This is usually assessed regularly during and before weight loss treatment. This is because fat existing in the lower body region is associated with higher health risks as compared

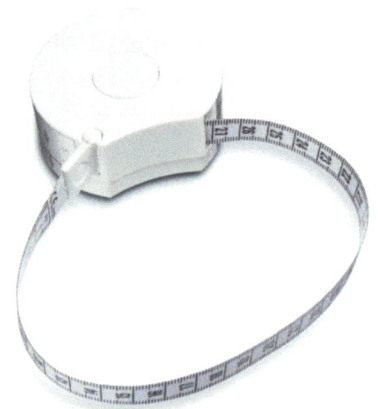

By: Oliver Greene

to peripheral fat.

Moreover, it is the abdominal fat that possesses independent health risks, even if the BMI does not indicate overweight or obesity. Therefore, both BMI and abdominal circumference should be measured in order to conduct the initial assessment of obesity as well as for monitoring the efficacy of the weight loss treatment.

Did You Know?
A high waist circumference is independently associated with high risk of hypertension, dylipidemia, diabetes, and CVD. People with BMI between 25 and 34.9 Kg/m2 are highly susceptible to such diseases.

High-Risk Waist Circumference

Men: >40 inch (>102 cm)

Women: >35 inch (>88 cm)

Although BMI and waist circumference are interrelated, the independent risk prediction of waist circumference that of BMI.

There are age related and ethnic differences when it comes to fat distribution in the body that modifies the predictive validity of waist circumference as a surrogate for abdominal fat. For elderly individuals, whose muscle loss is not taken into account by BMI, waist circumference assumes greater value in estimating the risks of obesity related diseases.

By: Oliver Greene

Causes of the Growing Epidemic

The prevalence of obesity is directly associated with the emergence of modern lifestyles throughout the world. In the light of scientific research, obesity occurs when a person consumes a greater number of calories than he or she burns. However, the causes of the imbalance of calories vary from person to person. Environmental, genetic, psychological, and many other factors play an active role in causing obesity.

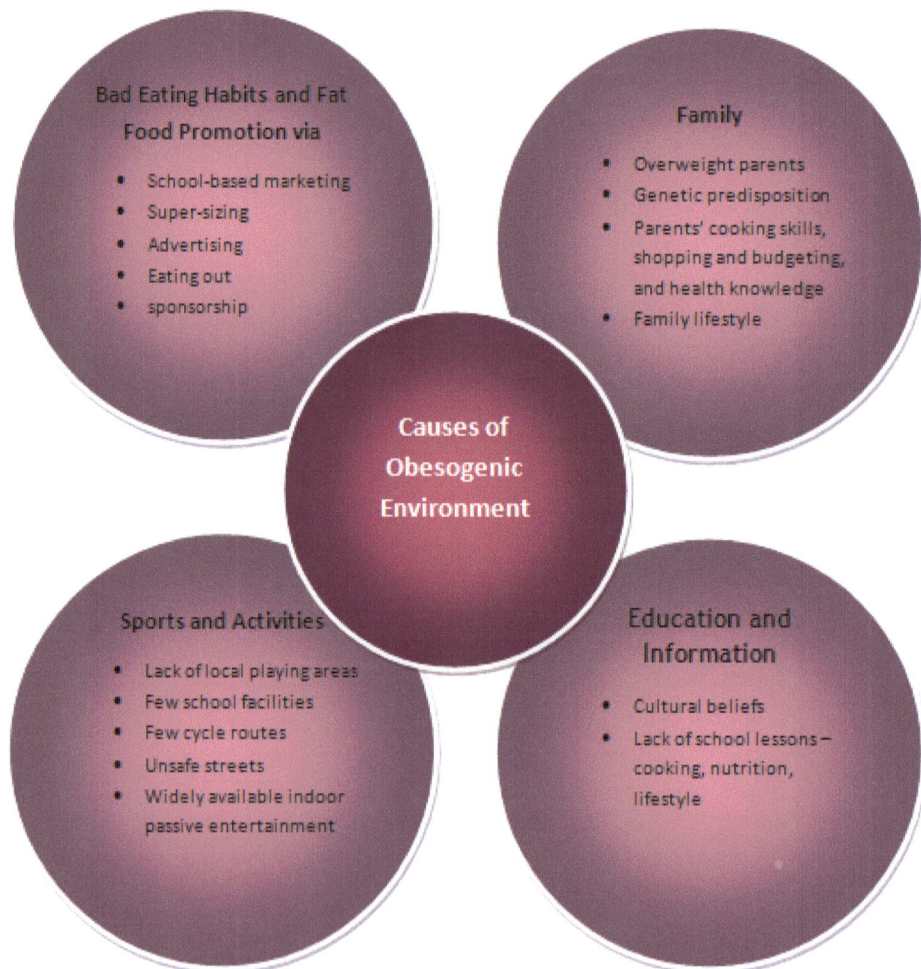

Bad Eating Habits and Fat Food Promotion via

- School-based marketing
- Super-sizing
- Advertising
- Eating out
- sponsorship

Family

- Overweight parents
- Genetic predisposition
- Parents' cooking skills, shopping and budgeting, and health knowledge
- Family lifestyle

Causes of Obesogenic Environment

Sports and Activities

- Lack of local playing areas
- Few school facilities
- Few cycle routes
- Unsafe streets
- Widely available indoor passive entertainment

Education and Information

- Cultural beliefs
- Lack of school lessons – cooking, nutrition, lifestyle

By: Oliver Greene

Environmental factors

Genes may not destine people to a lifetime of obesity, but lifestyle does. Environmental factors strongly influence obesity. This includes two very important aspects, the eating habits, and the level of physical activity. In a nutshell, it is the bad lifestyle of a person that leads to obesity and its health hazards.

People throughout the world are enjoying their convenient lifestyle and eating high-fat food, which is easily available. People nowadays are keeping taste ahead of nutrition and eating junk and fat-rich foods. And since everything is just a call or click away, they do not get enough physical activity.

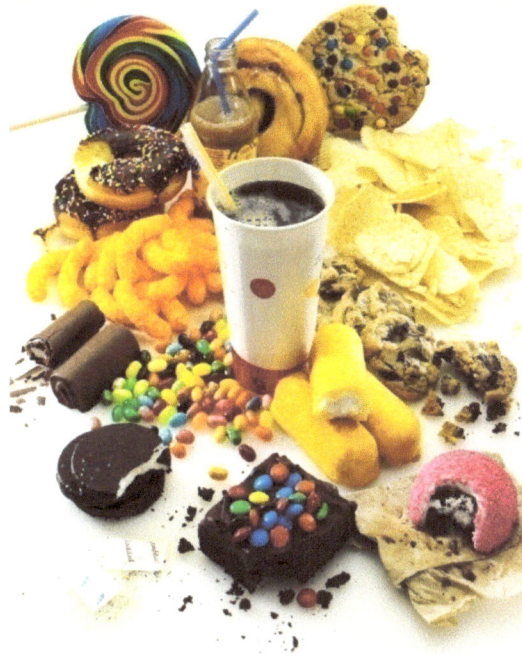

While genetic makeup could not be changed, there are some things that you can easily alter, which will have a very positive impact on your life. The first two things that desperately need a change are your eating habits and level of activities. The following are some easy techniques that can help you reduce and maintain weight:

- Prefer nutrition over taste and look for food that is more nutritious and low in fat.

By: Oliver Greene

- Learn to control and recognize environmental cues (for example, inviting smells) that trigger the craving to eat in you, even when you are not hungry.

- Become more active and do all housework by yourself. Use less cell phone and internet; instead walk down to the store to buy stuff yourself. Whenever possible, use stairs for climbing instead of the elevator or escalator.

- Maintain a timetable to keep records of your physical activity and food intake.

Genetic Factor

Obesity is a trend that tends to run in families. Obesity caused because of genes is referred to as genetic obesity. However, sometimes it is not only the genetic factor behind obesity; families tend to share lifestyle habits and diets that can contribute to excessive weight or obesity. This is why it often gets difficult to separate such factors from the genetic factors. Even so, according to science, obesity is strongly linked to heredity.

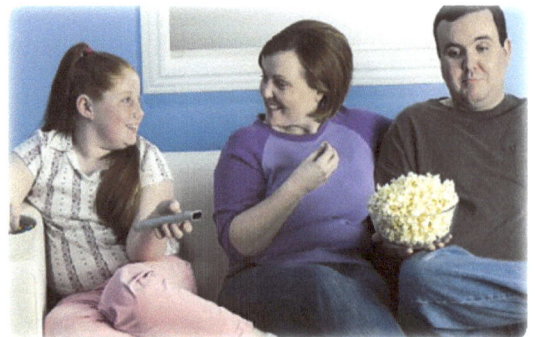

According to a study, adults who were adopted as children were found to have weights closer to their adoptive parents than their biological parents. In this case it is clear how lifestyle was more influential than genetic makeup.

By: Oliver Greene

Psychological Factors

Psychological factors also play a very influential role on the lifestyle of an individual. Many times, people eat more as a response to certain negative emotions such as anger, sadness, or boredom.

In addition, most overweight people tend to go through a more psychologically tough time than other average weight people. This is why many obese and overweight people suffer eating disorders when they try to reduce weight. People who are severely obese experience this disorder more commonly.

This eating disorder is very unhealthy and dangerous for people who are already overweight or obese. During the disorder episode, people eat large amounts of food recklessly without controlling how much they eat. Those with the most severe binge eating problems are also likely to have

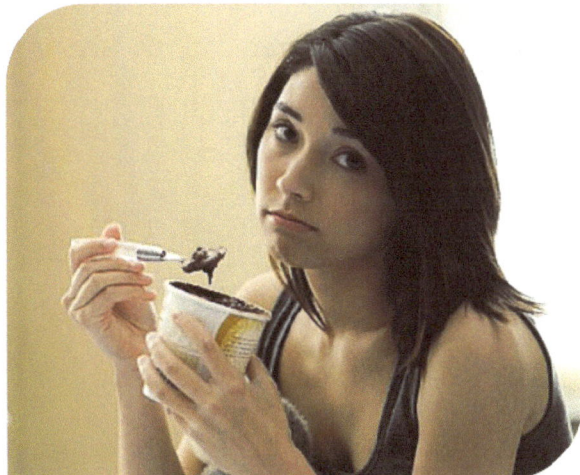

symptoms of low self-esteem and depression. Such people may even find it more difficult to reduce weight and keeping it off than people without the eating disorder problem.

If you have identified your binge eating problem, immediately seek help from a medical professional such as a clinical social worker, psychologist, or psychiatrist.

By: Oliver Greene

Other Obesity Causes

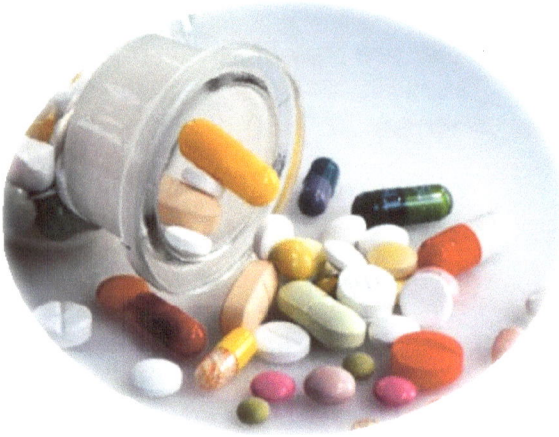

Certain medical conditions or illnesses increase the tendency to gain weight and lead to obesity. These include depression, Cushing's syndrome, hypothyroidism, and other neurological problems that can lead to various eating disorders. Also, steroids and other antidepressant drugs may cause weight gain. Therefore, it is very important to seek medical assistance before consuming such medication. Only a doctor can tell whether certain medical conditions and medications are underlying factors that causes weight gain or make weight loss difficult.

Consequences of Obesity

Obesity is not just a cosmetic problem – it is a health hazard. Around 300,000 adult deaths taking place every year in the United States are caused by obesity. There are many serious medical health conditions associated with obesity and excess weight. These include stroke, hypertension, heart disease, and type II diabetes. Overweight and obesity is also linked to certain types of cancer. Most obese men die from prostate cancer, rectum cancer, or colon cancer whereas obese women usually die from cancer of ovaries, cervix, uterus, breast, and gallbladder.

By: Oliver Greene

Other health problems and diseases associated to obesity include:

- Liver disease
- Gallstones and gallbladder disease
- Osteoarthritis – This is a disease of the bones in which the joints deteriorate. When excess weight is carried by joints, it usually results in osteoarthritis.
- Gout – Another joint disease caused by excess weight.
- Pulmonary problems – Breathing problems, including sleep apnea in which a person is unable to breath for a short while, while sleeping.
- Infertility and reproductive problems (in women) – Also leads to menstrual irregularities.

According to heath practitioners, the severity of health problems varies according to the severity of obesity. The more obese a person, the more likely he or she is to develop health problems.

Social and Psychological Effects

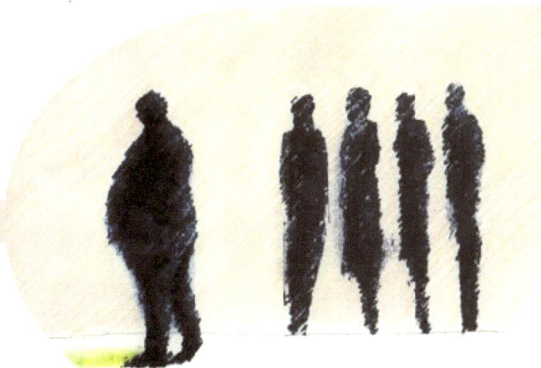

People think obese people are lazy, gluttonous, or both. While this may not be the case with most obese people, they still face discrimination or prejudice in social situations, at school, and in the job market. Feelings of depression, shame, or rejection are common.

By: Oliver Greene

So Who Should Reduce Weight?

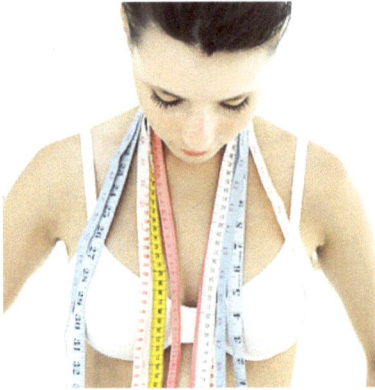

According to health care providers, people who have their Body Mass Index of equal to or higher than 30 must reduce weight and improve their health condition. This is specifically applicable on people who are severely obese.

The most painful part of being obese is the emotional suffering a person goes through. Many societies emphasizes on the importance of physical appearance and usually associate slimness with attractiveness, especially for women. Such customs make overweight and obese feel uncomfortable and unattractive. It is highly recommended to prevent additional weight gain if the BMI is between 25 and 29.9, unless there is susceptibility to other risk factors. It is recommended by obesity experts that a person must lose weight if they have two or more of the following:

- **Family history** – If there had been a family history of certain chronic disease, such as diabetes or heart disease, there is likelihood of you developing such problems if you get overweight or obese.
- **Pre-existing health condition** – High blood sugar levels, high cholesterol levels, or high blood pressure are all warning signs of some obesity-related diseases.
- **Body Shape –** People with 'apple shape' bodies are at a higher risk of developing diabetes, heart disease, or cancer as compared to people with a 'pear shape' body. This is because people with 'apple shape' body have their weight concentrated around their waist.

By: Oliver Greene

Obesity and the Risk Status

There are still many people in society who take their obesity and excess weight problem very casually. This is maybe because they are used to the way they are discriminated or treated in society or maybe because they haven't yet faced any medical consequences.

However, obesity is not a joke or a matter that can easily be overlooked. The medical consequences can be more severe than a person may expect. The bigger problem occurs when families as a whole get caught in the cyclone of obesity. Parents who have lived their lives being obese are not much concerned if their children are following the same path.

The following are the health consequences of obesity in detail, which can be used as eye-openers for parents and individuals.

Premature Death

- Approximately 300,000 deaths per year may be attributable to obesity.
- Death risks rise with increase in weight.
- Even if excess weight is moderate and falls between ten and twenty pounds, it increases the risk of death, particularly for people between the age of thirty and sixty-five years.
- In comparison with healthy weight people, individuals who are obese are susceptible of premature deaths from all causes.

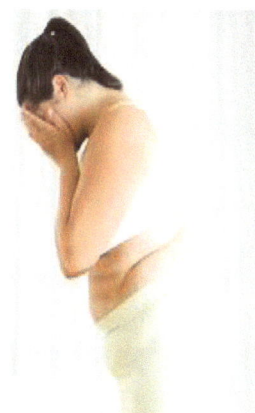

By: Oliver Greene

Diabetes

- If a person gains eleven to eighteen pounds of weight over their healthy weight, they become prone to the risk of developing type II diabetes, which is twice to that of individuals who maintain their healthy weight.

- More than 80 percent of people with diabetes are either obese or overweight.

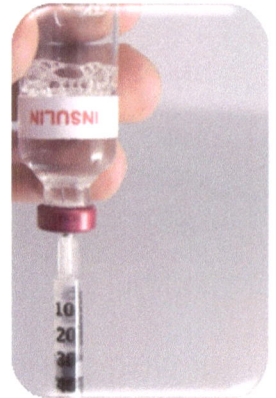

Heart Disease

- People who are obese or overweight increase the risk of various heart diseases such as heart attack, abnormal heart rhythm, chest pain or angina, sudden cardiac death, and congestive heart failure.

- Hypertension or high blood pressure is twice more common in obese adults than in those individuals who maintain healthy weight.

- High level of blood fat (triglycerides) and low level of HDL cholesterol (good cholesterol) is associated with obesity.

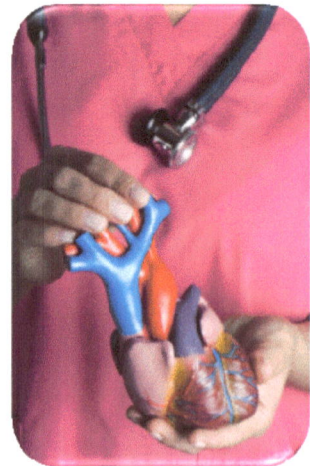

Cancer

- Obesity and excess weight are linked with high risk of certain types of cancer, including kidney, prostate, gall bladder, colon, endometrial, and postmenopausal breast cancer.

By: Oliver Greene

- Women who gain 20 excessive pounds in their late teenage to midlife increase the risk to double of developing postmenopausal breast cancer.

Breathing Problems

- Interrupted breathing during sleep or sleep apnea is a very common medical condition in obese people.
- Obesity is linked to a higher prevalence of asthma.

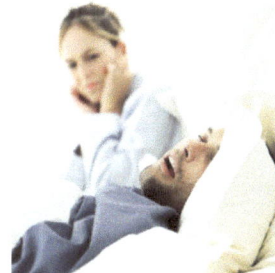

Arthritis

- With every additional increase of 2 pounds in weight, developing arthritis risk increases by 9 to 13 percent.
- Osteoarthritis is the most common arthritis type among obese people.

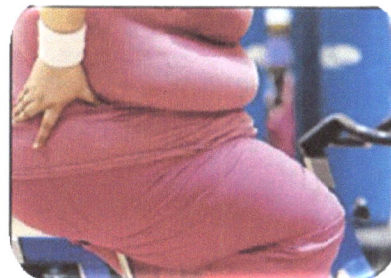

Additional Health Consequences

- Obesity and excess weight are associated with increased risks of incontinence, gall bladder disease, depression, and increased surgical risk.
- Obesity leads to limited mobility, which can further affect the quality of life. Moreover, it can result in decreased physical endurance through academic, social, and job discrimination.

People today must understand the menace of obesity and its deadly health consequences. They should realize that the primary concern of excess weight and obesity is one of health and not appearance.

By: Oliver Greene

The Risk Cycle

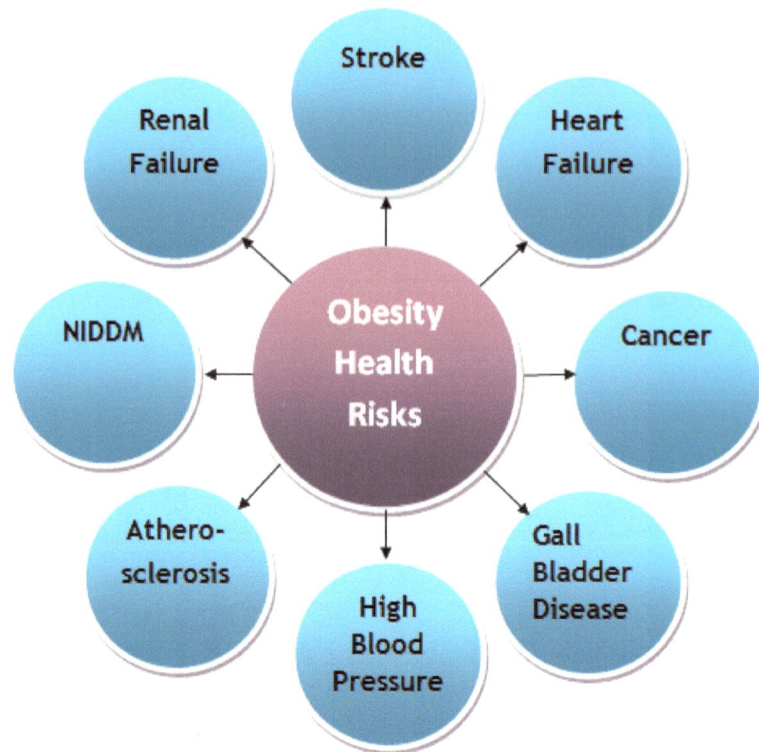

Stroke

Renal Failure

Heart Failure

NIDDM

Obesity Health Risks

Cancer

Athero-sclerosis

High Blood Pressure

Gall Bladder Disease

If you are obese, it is very important to realize your health risks. Drawn above is a 'Obesity Health Risks' cycle, which indicates the common health risks associated to obesity. Overweight or obese people, who have unhealthy eating and activity habits, have a higher risk of developing these severe health conditions.

This is also applicable for obese children, who are at the same risk for many of the long term health problems. In fact, a recent study revealed that the negative health consequences of obesity are far more distressing than health consequences that are associated with poverty, drinking, or smoking.

By: Oliver Greene

According to another study that took place in the United States, obesity affects more people than poverty, drinking, or smoking individually does in the US. This was confirmed by the statistics that showed an estimated of 23% people in the US who are obese, and 36% people who are overweight. This was a much higher rate when contrasted with 14% people living in poverty, 19 percent smokers, and only 6% heavy drinkers.

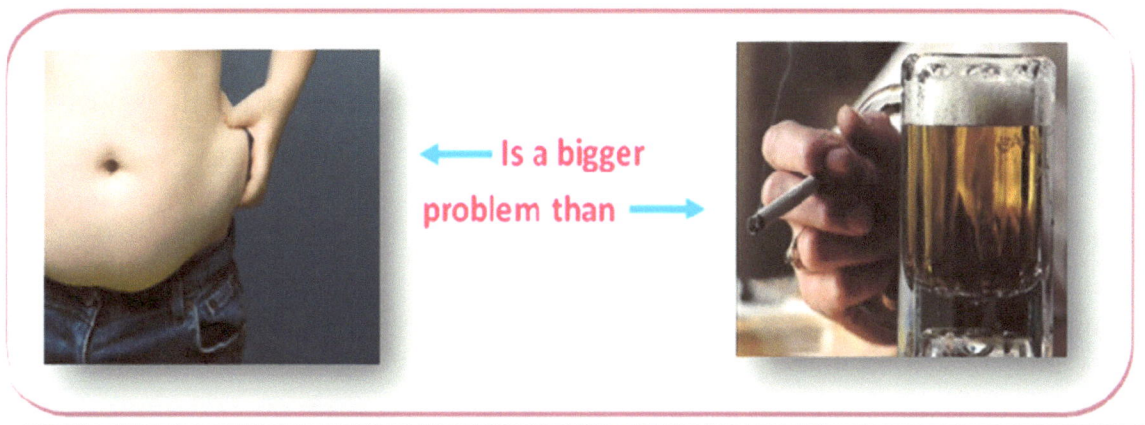

Obesity rates are dramatically increasing and thus increasing the obesity health risks for overweight and obese people. The lifestyle change has been very significant over the past 20 years. People all over the world are exercising less while maintaining or increasing the calorific intake.

There had also been a drastic increase in the number of fast food chains during the past few decades that are constantly forcing children and adults to eat unhealthy, sugary, and fatty food and sacrifice their health for

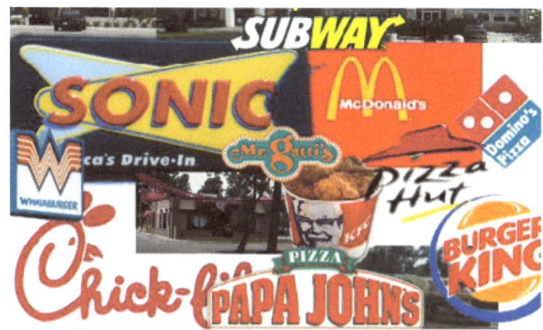

By: Oliver Greene

taste.

Increase in the number of hours devoted to watching television, desk jobs, and car-friendly modernized environments are some of the environmental changes that have contributed towards discouraging physical activity and encouraging intake of unhealthy fatty food.

These technological and environmental changes have not only affected the United States, but have also affected many other industrialized countries. For example, Germany and Great Britain have been experiencing similar obesity growth rates for the past 20 years. However, the only reason they have not yet reached an epidemic level like the US is because they started off with lower levels.

Obesity is a threat for not one country or two, but our planet as a whole.

Read on to find out the obesity health risks for women!

Female Obesity and Risk Factors

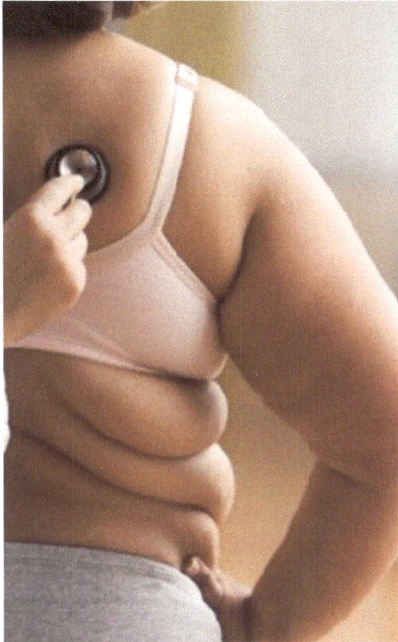

Obesity can have an adverse impact on health at each stage of a woman's life cycle. When young, obesity impacts the psychosocial health of women. However, as they grow older and become parents, they can experience bad reproductive health. Obesity also leads to pregnancy complications and imposes serious risks. In older women, obesity is linked to the emergence of a number of related chronic diseases, such as cardiovascular disease, type II diabetes, and increase risk for many types of cancers.

In short, obese women suffer more than others in terms of quality of life. With the growing health consequences of obesity, it is clear how obesity has a marked impact on life expectancy. But as far as female obesity is concerned, the medical risks associated are very important to identify and prevent since this keeps future generation at stake as well.

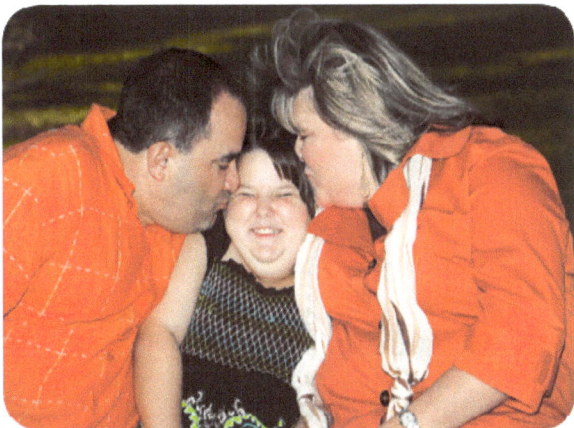

One obese woman can have a greater impact on the entire family than other obese individuals. If a woman is fit and healthy, she tends to keep the entire family healthy. On the other hand, an obese woman who has spent her entire life being overweight does not tend to pay much

By: Oliver Greene

attention to the lifestyle and health of her children. Eventually, the entire family becomes obese.

More often than not, it's obese mother who produce obese kids. Whether a mother models the right or the wrong behavior is a very big factor in determining which weight path the kids will go down.

Other than the risk of turning the whole family obese, there are many medical consequences and risk factors associated with female obesity. The following are some factors that lead to female obesity.

- Smoker women are usually at risk of becoming obese. Other than this, women with a family history of obesity also tend to gain weight and become obese either in their childhood or as adults. Moreover, women who are night-shift-workers also tend to gain weight since it increases the tendency

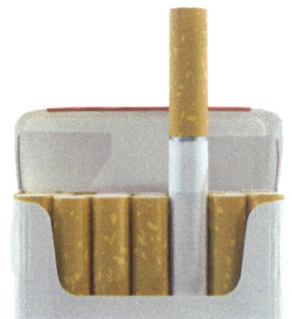

to snack more. Socioeconomic and ethnic factors also lead to female obesity – like Mexican Americans, African Americans etc.

- Menopause and pregnancy are also significant factors that contribute in the development of female obesity. This is caused by the fluctuations taking place in the reproductive hormone concentrations that uniquely predisposes women to gain excess weight.

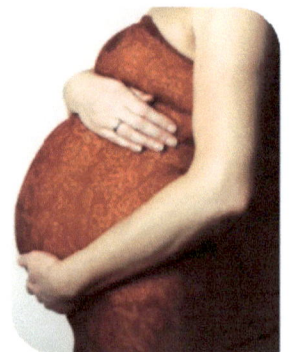

- Women with poor economic circumstances, fewer

By: Oliver Greene

years of education, and lower occupational status increases the risk of obesity.

@ Generally, women tend to have a high percentage of body fat as compared to men. This is the basic indication that women have lower basal fat oxidation thereby contributing to a higher fat storage.

Female obesity has increased by 15% over the past decade. According to studies, female obesity is fast becoming a dreaded factor around the world. Nearly 50% of all African American and Hispanic American women are overweight. As a result, they are becoming prone to many chronic diseases.

Female Obesity Symptoms

Female obesity can easily be judged by abnormal weight growth (body mass), which can also be measures by BMI (Body Mass Index). Apart from this obvious symptom, there are many other signs that witness female obesity. These include:

@ Lack of energy

@ Breathing problems

@ Disinterest in physical activities

@ Changes in the appearance

@ Pain in hips

@ Pain in knees and other joints

@ Pain in the back

Certain symptoms and signs of female obesity can be recognized by people on their own. However, there are other signs and symptoms that require a

By: Oliver Greene

professional doctor to diagnose. Female obesity symptoms that can easily be identified include:

- **Body Disproportion** – this is the most common symptom of obesity when one can easily feel the disproportion in different physical and facial features. Excess chin fat, cheek fat, and baby faces are typical of obese individuals.

- **Stretch Marks** – this is another very common symptom and obese individuals can easily see white or purple stretch marks appear around thighs and abdomen area.

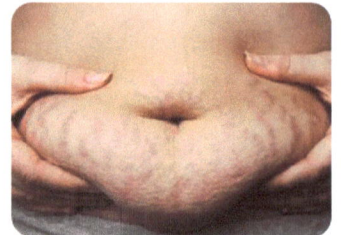

- **Thighs and Arms** – Fat cells usually cause thighs and arms to expand. This makes the thighs and arms to go saggy by losing the normal skin tightness.

- **Psychological Trauma** – people who are suffering obesity often experience increased stress, anxiety, and difficulties in accomplishing every-day ordinary tasks.

Obese women have become susceptible to all obesity related medical conditions. But the two most common problems that only obese women face are birth defects linked to obesity during pregnancy and breast cancer.

Reproductive Complications and Birth Defects

Obesity during pregnancy leads to increased risk of death in both the mother and the baby. This is because obesity during pregnancy tends to increase the blood pressure level of the mother by 10 times. In addition, obese women are more

By: Oliver Greene

likely to have gestational diabetes during pregnancy and later have problems with labor and delivery.

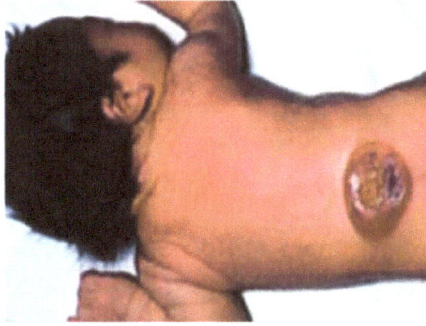

Studies have also linked obesity during pregnancy to several medical health conditions for both mothers and their offspring. Obese women expecting a baby go through an increased risk of birth defects, particularly neural tube defects, such as spina bifida and others like heart defects, brain defects, cleft palate, gastrointestinal defects, etc.

Female obesity increases the likelihood for pregnancy induced gestational diabetes, hypertension, cesarean delivery and other reproductive complications. Not only this, the newborns of obese mothers are at a higher risk for being overweight or obese and developing type II diabetes in later life.

Breast Cancer

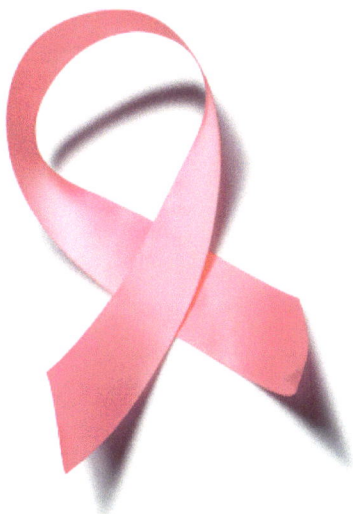

Breast cancer is the second most common cancer among women caused by obesity and several other factors. Obesity is among the most prominent factors of many other health conditions. It is said that healthy lifestyle choices can effectively protect women from developing this disease.

According to a women's health expert and clinical faculty member at New York Presbyterian hospital, cancer risks are present everywhere and are adopted

By: Oliver Greene

from everyday lifestyles. She insisted that the cancer risks include different factors out of which lifestyle choices are becoming a very prominent factor. Thus, simple changes made to ==your lifestyle== can easily help people reverse the risk of this deadly disease.

The following ==are a few== health related causes that leads to higher risk of breast cancer:

Overweight or obesity

Excessive weight is becoming the most common factor for breast cancer. If your weight is higher than it should be according to your height, you will be at a higher risk of developing this disease. Therefore, it is very important to prevent being overweight or obese especially after menopause, which experts believe may be due to changes in estrogen levels.

Sedentary lifestyle

Becoming a couch-potato and leading a sedentary lifestyle can efficiently contribute to an increased risk of developing breast cancer by adding excess weight as you grow older. Therefore, it is very important to combine healthy diet with regular exercise.

High fat diet

Eating high fat diet from your favorite junk food restaurant may also raise the risk of breast cancer. According to studies, there is a moderate link between dietary-fat intake and breast cancer. So, frequent stops at drive-through must be controlled in order to control the intake of high fat diet.

In a nutshell, reducing excessive weight is the only way women can prevent the increased risk of breast cancer and reproductive complications and birth defects.

Thus, a woman can reverse the obesity hazardous results from affecting the entire family if she wishes to. It is very much in control of a woman to prevent the epidemic from affecting her and her family.

Childhood Obesity

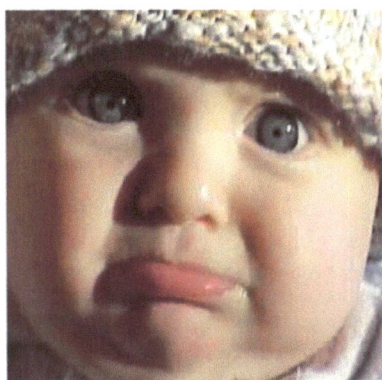

The prevalence of childhood obesity is dramatically rising at an alarming rate for several decades throughout the world. Childhood obesity has become a big threat to our world as a whole. It is indeed a very serious issue and has become a big matter of concern for the children of our nation.

Obesity can lead to various social and physical consequences and medical conditions that can destroy the childhood of any kid. Moreover, these consequences are often carried to adulthood, which affects the entire life of a person. This is why it is very important that we prevent and stop the growing epidemic and save our children from this menace.

Surprisingly, many parents are not even aware if their children are obese or overweight or are suffering from any health risks of carrying excess weight.

By: Oliver Greene

Parents who are obese themselves and have lived similar lives to that of their children tend to do this mistake more commonly. Parents who are food-lovers and are spending sedentary lifestyles fail to discourage their children from following a bad lifestyle or gaining more weight.

Even if parents are obese, they have no right to destroy their child's life by providing them a bad lifestyle that leads to obesity. No parent would want to deliberately let their child suffer the health risks and psychological consequences of being overweight or obese. Therefore, it is very important to identify and accept that your child is overweight if you really want to save him or her from the threats of excess weight.

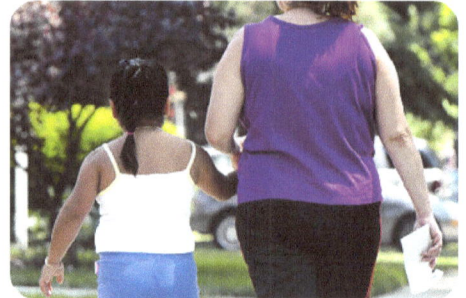

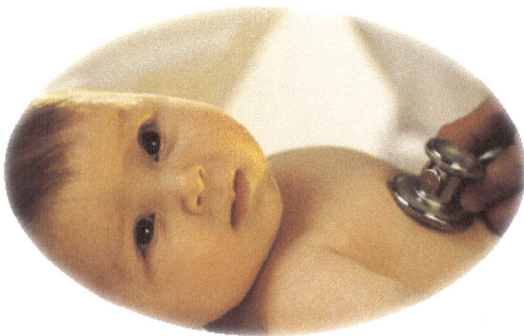

Childhood obesity has severe health risks. Sleep apnea, hypertension, type 2 diabetes, asthma, depression, and orthopedic compilation are some common health consequences that obese children are prone to. While all other emotional and psychological consequences can be overlooked, health risk is one major factor that no parent can ignore.

Just as the level of obesity gets severe in your child, the common diseases mentioned above will also get severe. Children suffering high level of

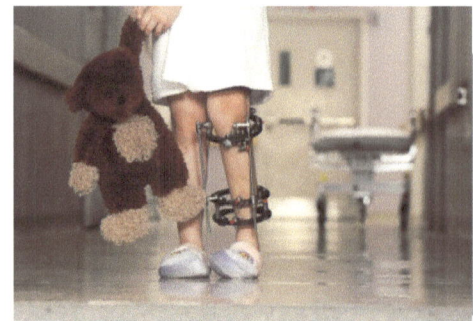

By: Oliver Greene

obesity become susceptible to dangerous diseases such as heart related diseases, joint and bone problems, high cholesterol, gall bladder and liver disease, and even cancer.

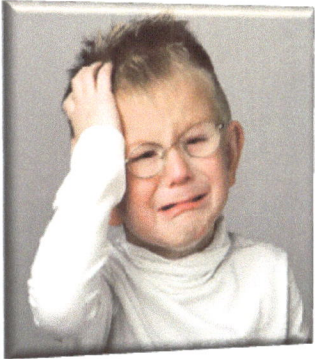

Apart from this, obese children who are unhappy about their excessive weight also get psychologically sensitive. They tend to develop eating disorders and substance abuse problems. If the threat of obesity in children is diagnosed and treated at an early stage, parents can save their children from going through such severe consequences.

Low self-esteem is another common mental condition that obese children face. This feeling grows especially when obese children are compared and discriminated with their non-obese friends and classmates. Research has revealed that an obese teenager who is going through psychological and self-esteem difficulties is more likely to start smoking and drinking alcohol. This is the main reason why children's lifestyle issues should mainly be focused on in order to control excessive weight or any other inappropriate behavioral change instead of imposing strict diets and calorie count.

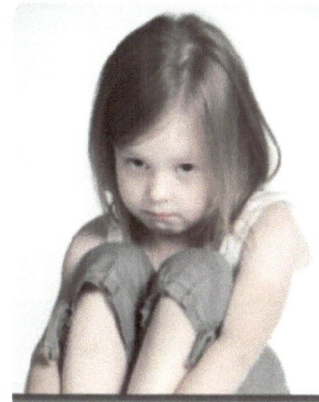

Childhood Obesity Causes

One thing that every parent must know is whether their child is overweight or is suffering obesity. There are several factors that lead to childhood obesity. Some major ones are as follows:

- **Food Marketing -** Fast food marketing is a primary culprit that attacks your children when you are not attentive. It is playing a very significant role in costing your child his or her health. These fast food companies are targeting young children and teenagers with their not-so healthy food advertisements. It is not the mistake of an individual if he or she is getting attracted to this advertisement since

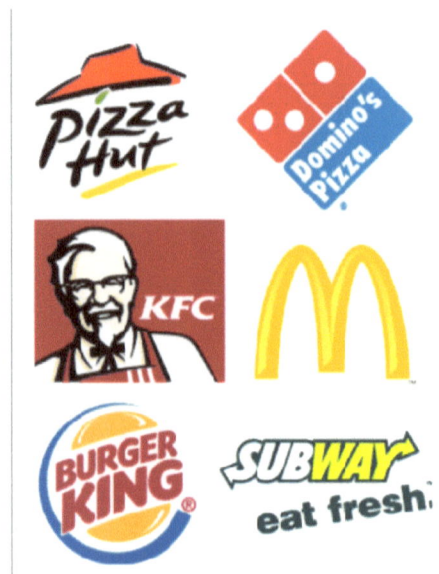

they are indeed very interesting and eye-catching. Although there is not much parents can do about these advertisements, cutting down the screen time for your children can save them from the exposure of these tempting fast food advertisements.

- **Bad Eating Habits –** Parents should accept that they are compromising on the dietary patterns and bad eating habits of their children. When a kid asks for a high-fat meal from a restaurant, it is very rare to see any parent turn down the request. Other than this, parents themselves are

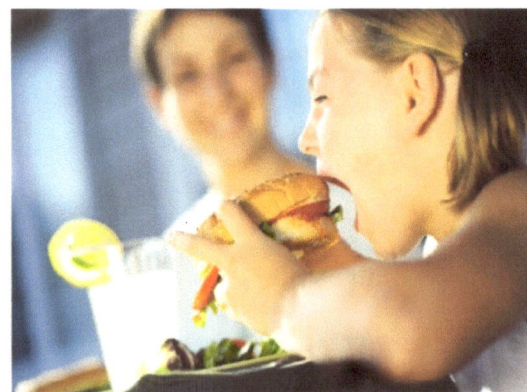

cooking high caloric food or depending on processed and unhealthy food from the market. Eating high calorie fattening food is one of the major reasons for childhood obesity.

By: Oliver Greene

- **Sedentary Lifestyle** – Undoubtedly, a sedentary lifestyle is the most obvious reason why children today are gaining weight and becoming obese. Media and technological advancement are playing a great role in making lives sedentary and

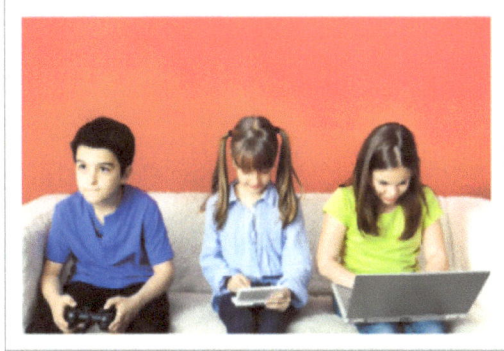

inactive. Children and adults are becoming couch potatoes and spending more and more time in front of televisions and laptops. Specifically, children are so fond of their online games and television games today that outdoor sport games does not seem to have any importance anymore.

- **Lifestyle at School** – Children spend most of the day at school and therefore tend to follow the behavior choices and lifestyle common in their schools. Thus, it is clear how important it is for schools to pay attention to the health of their students and prevent any activities that are contributing to

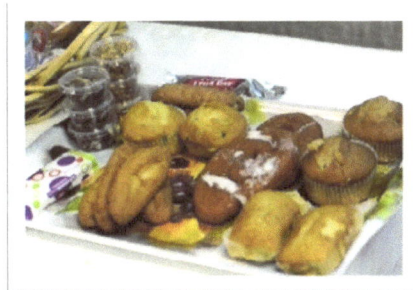

childhood obesity. This focuses mainly on the type of food provided in school, the physical activity options given to children, and educating children about the importance of maintaining health and preventing overweight and obesity.

- **Lifestyle at Home** – the behavioral pattern followed in a house related to eating habits, exercising and physical activity, shopping, and cooking play a major role in maintaining the balance of energy in the life of their children.

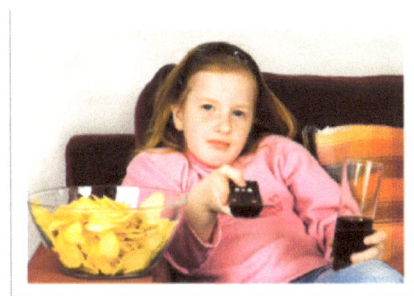

By: Oliver Greene

The entire lifestyle at home should be healthy in order to encourage children to adopt a healthy and risk-free lifestyle.

Parents cannot blame the children completely if they are fond of sweet and fatty food, since even parents know that such type of food is very enticing and tasty. However, it is strange to see how the life expectancy of our children has become lower than our own. Blaming one factor may not be appropriate since all the factors leading to obesity are associated with each other.

One cannot deny that the genetic factor is one of the major reasons for childhood obesity but environmental factors cannot be overlooked either. Apart from this, food marketing is another major reason why children are adopting bad eating habits and gaining weight.

What Can Parents Do To Help Children Fight Obesity?

Parents can:

- Help children incorporate physical activity in their daily routine.
- Encourage their children to eat healthy and nutritious foods by preparing healthy food at home and avoid regular restaurant trips and stops at drive-through.

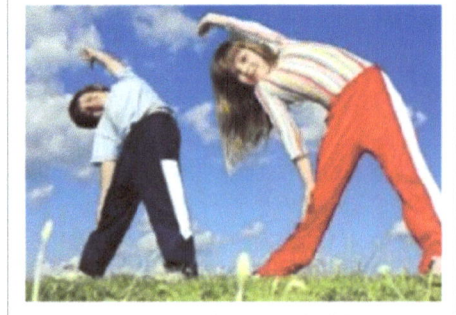

- Discourage children from consuming large portion sizes of the meal.
- Dedicate sweet treat and/or high-calorie food strictly for special days and occasions.

By: Oliver Greene

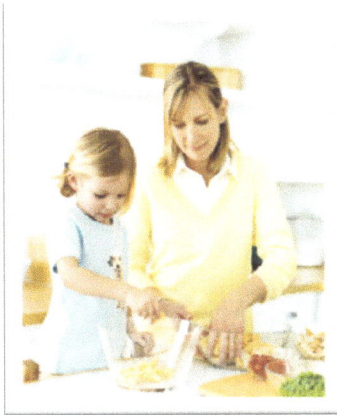

- Help children engage in physical activities by letting them help in kitchen or other work at home.

- Help children learn the benefits of healthy eating and active lifestyle and the drawbacks and health consequences related to obesity.

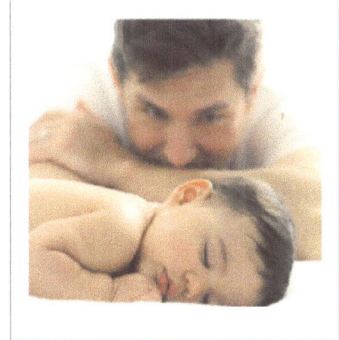

- Set appropriate sleeping routine for their children to make sure they are getting adequate sleep as it can help reduce the risk of obesity.

- Limit the time for each activity for children and make their daily time table more productive and contributing towards a healthy lifestyle.

- Limit the screen time and encourage children to participate in outdoor sports that promote physical activity.

- Give access to more milk and water to children instead of sodas, fruit juices, and soft drinks.

- Activate physical activity time for the entire family after dinner, which can help the family members digest the food well change the calories into energy before bedtime.

- Become a role model for their children and they can follow the same lifestyle to help their children adopt a healthy behavior towards eating and exercising.

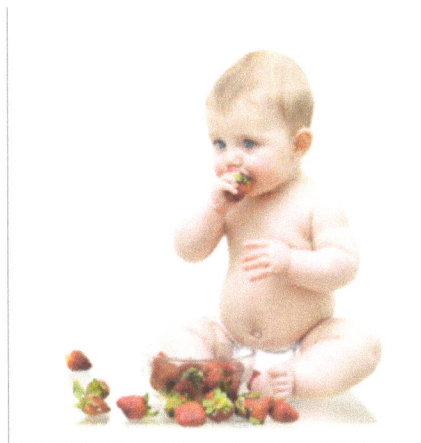

By: Oliver Greene

Both diet and exercise adds to the healthy lifestyle of your children. In order to be healthy, a child must follow healthy eating habits and an active lifestyle. This is where the role of parents comes in.

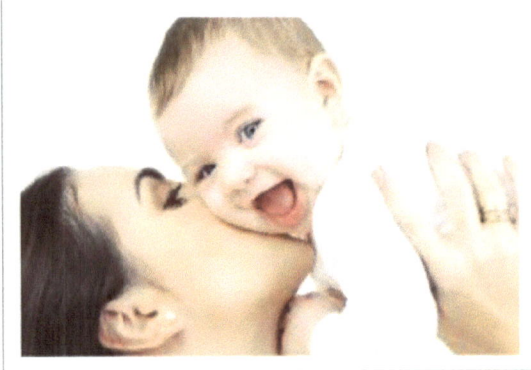

Parents play the role model in their children's life. Only you can change the lifestyle for your children and the entire family. It is the parents who can actually put efforts to fight childhood obesity on behalf of their children. Therefore, it is very important to target a goal and construct a plan. It is way easier to encourage children to adopt a new lifestyle as compared to adults.

Do not hesitate to turn down any wish or desire that takes them closer to the risk of childhood obesity. Today, they may fail to understand you, but tomorrow they will thank you for the justice you did to them and their health.

By: Oliver Greene

Evaluation and Treatment

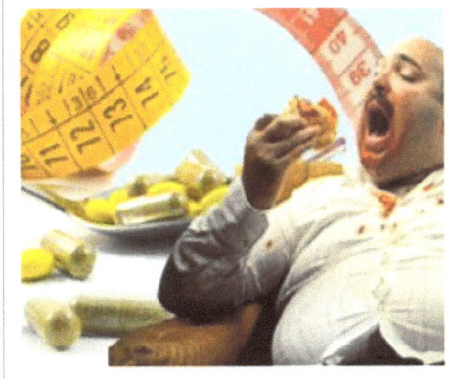

Evaluating the severity of obesity and treating it is very important. Not only because it is a growing epidemic, but also because it is a life-threatening disease associated with many health-risk factors. Obesity must be taken into account as it is actually a sign of what may well be a spectrum of different kinds of disorders – environmental and genetic.

Although obesity in itself is associated with increased risk of mortality and morbidity, poorly monitored and massive weight loss cycle can result in similarly dire consequences. The potential complications that are to be watched out during the weight loss cycle include electrolyte derangements, cardiac arrhythmias, hyperuricemia, hypokalemia, and psychological sequel, including eating disorders and depression.

In addition, the clear assessment of the person's level of motivation related to the exercise, dietary, and behavioral changes required to maintain weight loss is essential. This assessment should be conducted before any weight loss program or therapy is planned. It requires an informed, written, and comprehensive consent to concentrate on the required changes and expected weight loss.

Since weight loss attempt for obese individuals incorporates potential harm for unsuitable candidates, all the obese patients enrolled in any medical, surgical, or

By: Oliver Greene

other weight-loss programs requires exhaustive screening for underlying psychologic, psychiatric, or eating disorders.

In treating obesity, it is very important for the obese individuals to understand what they actually need to accomplish. Getting specific with their goal will increase their chances of achieving it rather than focusing on a general goal. Moreover, an obese individual should seek a goal that is **SMART**.

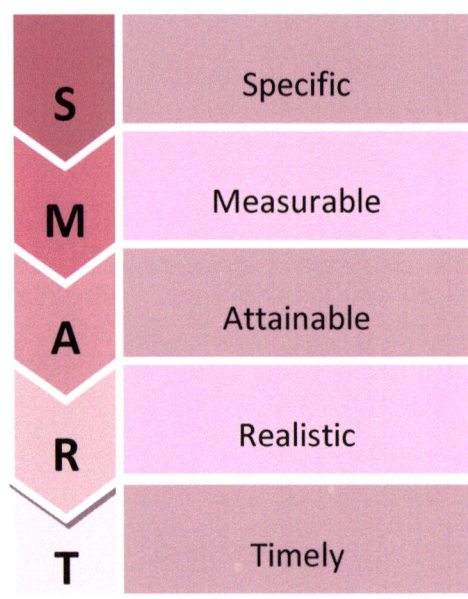

S	Specific
M	Measurable
A	Attainable
R	Realistic
T	Timely

Following a SMART goal helps individuals stick to it for a longer period and experience quick and positive results.

Another major factor that obese people must consider is culturally adapted weight-loss program. Every weight loss program is not suitable for all obese people. This is why culturally adapted weight loss program is considered an important and reasonable weight loss goal. The weight of the individual must be compared against the family's weight, ethnicity, culture, and racial background. This helps in setting individualized weight loss goals.

Obesity Treatment and Its Connection to Lifestyle

Lifestyle is rigorously connected to obesity treatment. Unless a person is willing to change his or her lifestyle, the weight loss goal cannot be accomplished. There are some strategies obese people must incorporate in their lifestyles in order to be successful. To overcome obesity, you must make the following additions to your obesity treatment plan.

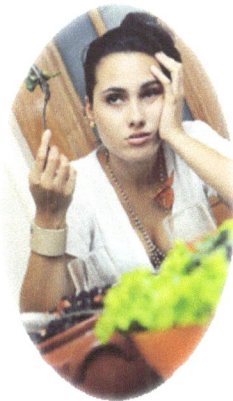

- **Treatment plan** – It is not easy for anyone to adopt a completely new lifestyle dramatically. Lifestyle that people stick to for many years is not easy to quit at once. No matter which weight loss program you follow, be honest with your health care providers, therapists or doctors. Do not hesitate to accept if you eating goals and activities are slipping off your hand. You may not be able to help it on your own, but together with the help of a health care provider, you can come up with new approaches and ideas that will help you get back in your new routine.

- **Medications** – In case you are taking any medication for weight loss or for treating conditions caused by obesity, such as diabetes or hypertension, take them exactly as prescribed by the doctor. If you face any trouble or unpleasant side effects of your medication regimen, visit your doctor and discuss your problem.

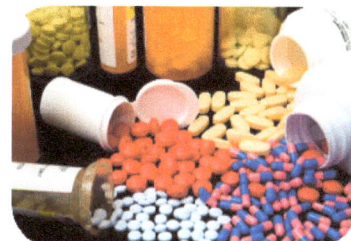

By: Oliver Greene

@ **Educate Yourself –** It is very important that you learn about your own condition. The more knowledge you have about obesity, the better you will know why you became obese and what measures you can take to overcome it. Once you learn about the health consequences of obesity, you will take this disease seriously and will be more determined to stick to your weight loss program and treatment plan. Read books, surf the internet, or talk to your therapist or doctor about it.

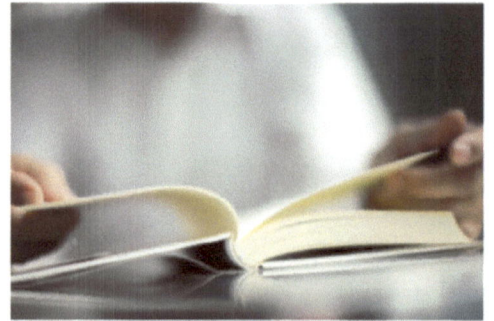

@ **Support –** It is almost impossible to achieve weight loss goals without a support. Get your friends and family on board and persuade them to support you at each and every step. Make sure your loved ones understand the importance of weight loss for your health. Apart from this, there are many weight loss support groups that you can join to get the encouragement you need.

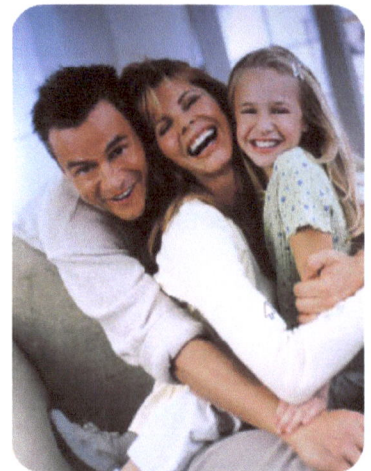

@ **Realistic Goals –** Do not be unrealistic with weight loss as obesity is a very serious problem. Setting goals such as reducing too much weight too fast is a very unrealistic approach. Do not set yourself up to face failure. Instead, set weekly or daily goals for weight loss and exercise. Start with a slow and gradual change and do not attempt to bring drastic changes to your diet. This approach is wrong and you are not likely to stick with for the long haul.

By: Oliver Greene

Food – food triggers must be identified and avoided. In short, distract yourself from food craving by engaging yourself with something else more positive, such as walking down the street to pick your children up from their piano class. Build up the courage to say 'NO' to big portions and unhealthy foods. Eat only when you actually feel hungry and not because its time to eat.

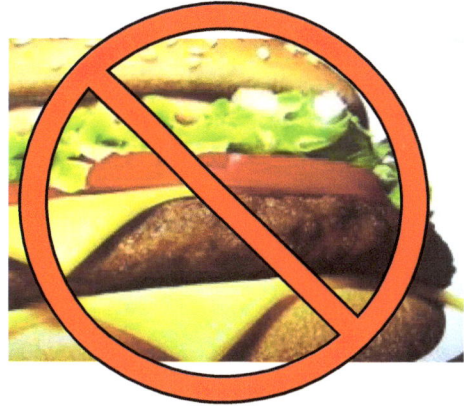

Record – maintain a journal to keep a record of activity and food consumed. This journal will help you stay accountable for your exercise and eating habits. This way it will become easier for you to see and identify the behavior that keeps holding you back. On the other hand, it will also let you learn about the behaviour that works well for you. Moreover, the journal will also help you track important health parameters such as cholesterol levels, blood pressure and overall health fitness.

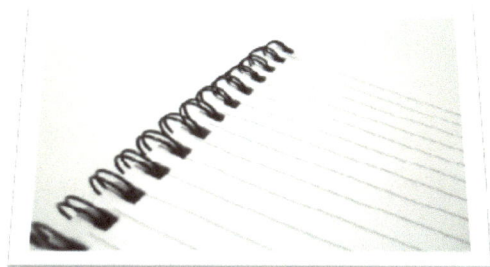

One thing that obese people should keep in their mind is that any treatment or program will take time to show results. No natural procedure or treatment can show dramatic and quick results. Therefore, it is very wise to keep patience and follow the treatment or weight loss program for a longer period instead of giving up with disappointment. Only a positive approach will give positive results.

By: Oliver Greene

The Facts about Obesity Treatment – Medication

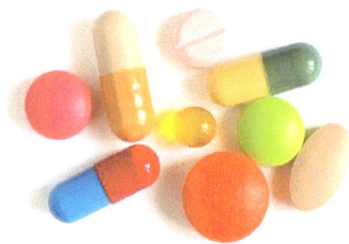

Although the best way to reduce weight is through a natural healthy diet and exercise program, in some situations these may not be the only advisable options. The third option for many people is weight-loss medication. However, one should not forget that weight-loss medication must be used alongside exercise, diet, and lifestyle changes for effective results. If the other factors are kept constant, medication is unlikely to work.

Doctors usually recommend the natural ways of reducing weight. Therapists and doctors mainly focus on your lifestyle changes, dietary patterns, and exercise routine to bring a decline in your weight. However, your doctor may prescribe weight loss medication if:

- Other weight loss methods aren't working for you.
- Your BMI has crossed 27 and you are suffering other obesity complications, such as sleep apnea, high blood pressure, and diabetes.

So if you are wondering whether weight-loss medication is the solution to overcome obesity, then read on to find out your answer.

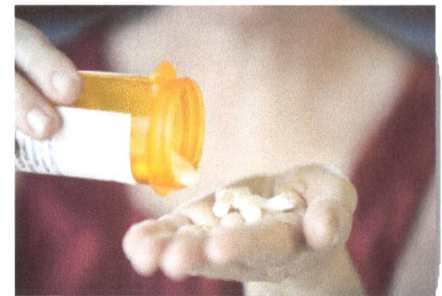

By: Oliver Greene

How Medicines Work to Help You Lose Weight?

It is basically the appetite suppressants that are considered effective in helping people to reduce weight.

- Appetite suppressants decrease appetite by increasing levels of catecholamines and serotonin. These are chemicals present in the brain that affect appetite and mood.

- Some medicines are considered effective as they work by disrupting the enzyme present in the intestines called lipase. This enzyme controls fat absorption. The medicine works to prevent 30% of the fat from digesting and absorbing. This fat is then excreted, which eventually lowers the calorie intake.

These medicines work only when in conjunction with change in lifestyle, eating patterns, and physical activity. According to a research study, obese people who increase physical activity, eat less, and take weight loss medication lose significantly more weight than people who follow medication without bringing any change to their lifestyle.

Like all drugs, medicines that are used to treat excess weight and obesity tend to have undesirable risks and powerful side effects.

Remember!

- Weight loss medications must only be used when prescribed by a medical professional, and only for people who are going through severe health problems related to obesity.

By: Oliver Greene

- These usually include people with a Body Mass Index of more than 27 and 30 and are highly susceptible to risk factors such as high cholesterol or high blood pressure.
- These medications are strictly not advisable for cosmetic or minor weight loss.

Traditional weight loss medication was only prescribed for a few months or weeks, but weight loss medication available today can be used for longer periods. However, studies are still going on to see how weight loss medication can result in long term side effects.

Pros and Cons of Weight loss Medication

The only possible and most desirable short term benefit of using weight loss medication is 'weight loss', which may help obese individuals lower the risk of certain health problems associated with obesity. However, its impact on an overall improvement in health over the long term is still unknown.

These medications are not without risks and include many side effects that may vary according to medicine.

- Side effects are a major concern for people who are only suffering from obesity and are healthy otherwise.
- Other concerns include the potential for abuse of the drugs.
- People relying on these drugs for weight loss usually experience that their weight loss tapers off after four to six months. This indicates that the medicine has reached its limit of effectiveness and is no longer effective.

By: Oliver Greene

To make sure these medicines are safe for your, consult your health care provider before taking any of these weight loss drugs. Let the medical professional tell you if you have any of the following medical conditions:

- High blood pressure
- Diabetes
- Glaucoma
- Eating disorder
- Heart disease or any other heart condition, like irregular heartbeat
- Drug, alcohol, or other substance abuse
- Bipolar disorder or depression
- Migraine
- Breastfeeding or pregnant

While the benefit is only one, there are several risk factors associated with using medication. It is not necessary to take medicines and drugs to control appetite and work abnormally with the enzymes and chemicals of the body. Behavioral therapy and determination towards changing lifestyle accordingly can also help people fight their appetite and craving for food.

It only needs a positive approach instead of taking a number of medicines that carry various side effects with them. So avoid this path and achieve natural weight loss as much as you can to be honest with your health.

By: Oliver Greene

Common Surgery Methods – Pros and Cons

It is not easy to decide if one should get weight loss surgery. And even after the decision is made, there are so many procedures to choose from. However, the most appropriate procedure for you depends on many things: your current health, the preference of your surgeon, your goals, and, of course, the procedures that are covered by your insurance, NHS or the system for surgery as covered in your respective country.

Although it requires a lot of discussion and thought before choosing the right weight-loss surgical approach, you must consider some basic information that will help you get started.

There are many surgical weight-loss procedures with several variations. The following is a general overview of surgical approaches that your doctor may recommend.

Adjustable Gastric Banding

Gastric banding is the least invasive weight loss treatment. In this surgery, the stomach is squeezed into two different sections with an inflatable band. The two sections include a smaller upper pouch and a lower section that is larger.

Although the stomach is squeezed into two sections, it is still

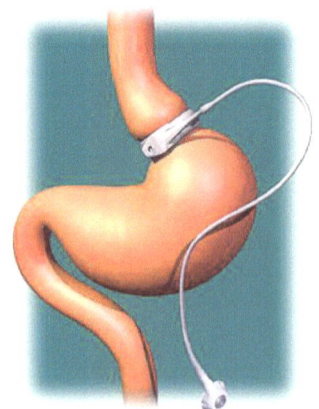

By: Oliver Greene

connected through a very narrow channel. This slows down the emptying of the upper pouch. This surgery effectively restricts the amount of food a person consumes. Since the upper pouch takes time to empty and is full with very little amount of food, a person is unable to eat more. Moreover, it requires the food to be well-chewed or soft.

Pros: Gastric banding is comparatively a simpler procedure and safer than other operations such as gastric bypass. It is a very common invasive surgery and includes special instruments, small incisions, and laparoscope (a tiny camera). Recovery of gastric banding surgery is usually fast and it can easily be reversed by removing the band surgically.

Since the band is adjustable and its opening is just beneath the abdominal skin, the band can be easily tightened or loosened by the doctor by increasing and decreasing the level of saline liquid, respectively.

Cons: Since gastric banding is a least invasive surgery, people usually experience less dramatic weight loss as compared to surgeries that are more invasive. Moreover, people who go through gastric banding are likely to regain weight over the years.

Risks: vomiting is the most common health consequence of gastric banding. It is usually caused by overeating too quickly. The band itself has many complications. It is very common that the band slips out of place, leak, or become loose. This requires further surgeries to fix the band back to its right place. Infections are always a big risk with surgeries. Although unlikely, certain complications can be life-threatening.

By: Oliver Greene

Sleeve Gastrectomy

It is comparatively a newer form of weight loss surgery. In sleeve gastrectomy operation around 75 percent of the stomach is removed. The remaining 25 percent of the stomach is basically a sleeve or a narrow tube that is connected to the intestines.

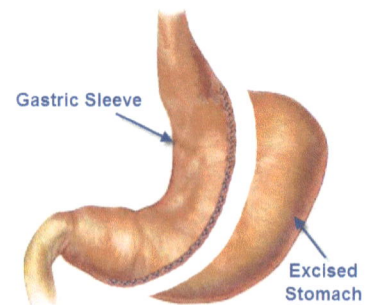

There is a sequence of weight loss surgeries in which sleeve gastrectomy is considered the first step. This step is usually followed by the next steps known as biliopancreatic diversion or gastric bypass. This is done in order to achieve greater weight loss.

Pros: For excessively sick or obese people, going directly for biliopancreatic diversion or standard gastric bypass can be very risky. Since sleeve gastrectomy is a relatively simpler surgery, it helps lowering the risk of other weight loss procedures. Later on, when a certain amount of weight loss is achieved and health is also improved, people can go for another surgery, such as gastric bypass.

Sleeve gastrectomy works as effectively as adjustable gastric banding, but since the intestines are not affected in sleeve gastrectomy surgery, the food absorption is not affected either. In short, sleeve gastrectomy is safer as it does not cause nutritional deficiencies.

Cons: Since sleeve gastrectomy surgery is the initial surgery for weight loss, there are other surgeries that you are to face later on. Another problem with this surgery is that it is irreversible. Once the part of stomach is removed, it can't be

By: Oliver Greene

joined back. And last but not the least, since it is a newer concept, the long term risks and benefits are not yet known.

Risks: Sleeve gastrectomy risks include typical surgical risks such as infection. Blood clots and leaking of the sleeve are other risks associated with this surgery.

Gastric Bypass Surgery

This is the most common weight loss surgery. This is one type of surgery that combines both malabsorptive and restrictive approaches. This surgery can be done as an open surgery or as minimally invasive.

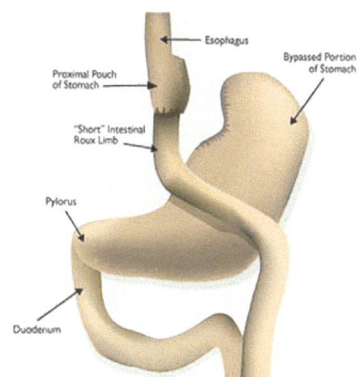

In gastric bypass surgery, the stomach is divided into two unconnected parts. The upper stomach is then directly connected to the small intestine. This is done in order to create a shortcut for food, bypassing small intestine and a section of the stomach. The purpose of skipping the lower part of the stomach during the digestion process is to get fewer calories absorbed into the body.

Pros: weight loss resulted from gastric bypass surgery tends to be dramatic and swift. Most of the weight loss is achieved during the first six months after the surgery. Moreover, it improves other health condition such as heartburn, sleep apnea, arthritis, high cholesterol, high blood pressure, diabetes, and other conditions caused by obesity. In a nutshell, people experience significant improvement in the quality of their life.

By: Oliver Greene

According to studies, gastric bypass has proven long term effectiveness and can keep their reduced weight off for ten years or more.

Cons: Surgeries like gastric bypass impair the ability of the body to absorb food. Although it can result in dramatic weight loss, it is full of many serious nutritional deficiencies risks. The loss of iron and calcium can lead to anemia and osteoporosis. People who choose this surgery should be very careful with their diet and must take additional supplements to counter the nutritional deficiencies.

Another problem of gastric bypass is the dumping syndrome. This is a syndrome in which food is quickly dumped in the intestines from the stomach without being properly digested. Dumping syndrome cases symptoms like diarrhea, weakness, sweating, pain, bloating, and nausea. Dumping syndrome is usually triggered by high-carbohydrate or sugary foods that leads to weight gain.

Risks: Gastric bypass is a relatively more complicated weight loss surgery and therefore is prone to higher risks. Although the risk of death from this surgery is very low, it is still more dangerous than many other types of weight loss surgeries, such as gastric banding. Blood clots and infections are also a major risk. Gastric bypass surgery also increases the risk of developing hernias, which needs further surgeries to get fixed.

Biliopancreatic Diversion

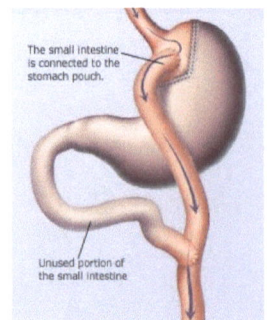

The small intestine is connected to the stomach pouch.

Unused portion of the small intestine

This surgery is a little less extreme version of gastric bypass weight loss surgery. Biliopancreatic diversion surgery includes a duodenal switch. Although it is much like gastric bypass, it involves removing less part of the stomach and bypasses less of

By: Oliver Greene

the small intestine. Moreover, it diminishes the risks of ulcers, malnutrition, and dumping syndrome, which are common with gastric bypass.

Pros: Biliopancreatic diversion has shown much faster and greater weight loss results as compared to gastric bypass. According to studies, this surgery can help a person loose around 75 to 80 percent of the excessive fat. Although a big section of the stomach is removed, the remaining is larger than the sections formed during banding procedures and gastric bypass. This way you can eat more food without feeling sick.

Cons: Although this weight loss surgery is very famous, it is less common than gastric bypass. This is because doctors do not recommend this surgery as the risks of nutritional deficiencies after this surgery are much higher and serious. Other than this, this surgery poses similar risks to that of gastric bypass including the severe dumping syndrome.

Risks: Biliopancreatic diversion is one of the most risky and complicated weight loss surgeries. This is one surgery that has the highest death rate probability ranging between 2.5 to 5 percent. As compared to gastric bypass, the risk of hernia after biliopancreatic diversion is fairly high.

Which is the best weight loss Surgery?

Your body type and your current health condition will help you determine the best weight loss surgery that is suitable for you. For instance, if you had already gone through an abdominal surgery before, or you are extremely obese, then going for a less invasive surgery may not be very effective

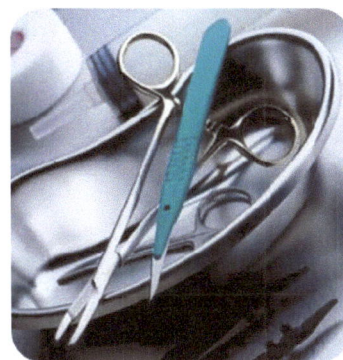

By: Oliver Greene

for you. Therefore, make sure you talk in detail with your doctor about the pros and cons of all the procedures.

Before deciding on the right surgery for you, it is advisable if you go to a medical center that specialized in weight loss therapies and surgeries. According to studies, the risks of weight loss surgeries are lower when handled by medical experts. No matter which region you belong to, make sure that you find yourself a well experienced surgeon to handle your obesity problem.

Is Weight Loss Surgery Right For Me?

While anybody can be obese, weight loss surgeries are not for everyone. These surgeries are only recommended for people who:

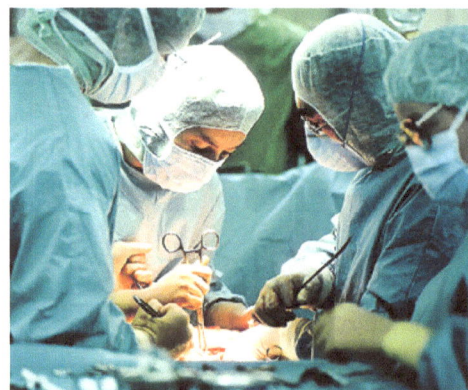

- Are suffering from severe obesity and have a BMI of 40 or more. This would be an excess of eighty pounds for women and one hundred pounds for men.
- Are not only obese (with BMI between 35 and 40) but are also suffering with serious health conditions of obesity, such as high cholesterol, sleep apnea, type 2 diabetes, heart disease, etc.
- Have tried but failed to lose weight naturally.
- Completely understand the risks.

The FDA has approved using Lap-Band surgery for individuals who have crossed the BMI of 30 and who are suffering at least one obesity-related health condition, such as high cholesterol.

By: Oliver Greene

Even if these basic criteria are met, there are many other factors one must consider. Perhaps, the most important part is to prepare yourself mentally. It can save the life of an obese individual to go through a successful weight loss surgery, but it is not a cure.

Instead, it is the first step in taking up a lifelong commitment. No surgery would be helpful on a long run basis until and unless you are ready to help yourself. Dedicate yourself to making permanent and dramatic changes to your lifestyle – how you eat, exercise, and live!

Obesity Management Techniques

By: Oliver Greene

Apart from drugs and surgeries, there are other obesity management techniques that involve natural therapies to help people change their lifestyle and achieve weight loss. While medication and surgeries can help obese individuals reduce weight dramatically, there is no guarantee that the weight loss is permanent. It is only the lifestyle of the person that can guarantee any permanent changes one wants to bring to his or her life.

The goal of obesity treatment is to achieve weight loss and maintain healthy weight forever. While you can always encourage yourself to incorporate positive changes in your lifestyle in order to reduce weight and live a healthy life, there are many other people who can help you accomplish your weight loss goal. A team of health professionals, including an obesity specialist, a therapist, dietitian, and a nutritionist can help your understand and make changes to your diet, activity habits, and behavior.

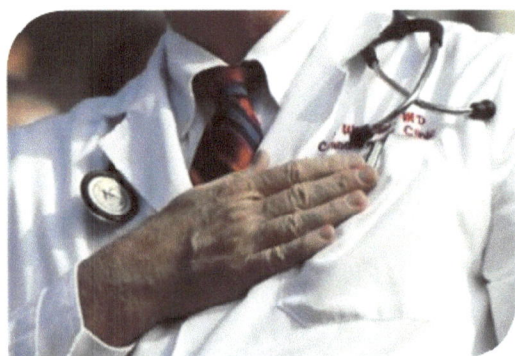

Treatment for weight loss methods that are suitable for you will depend on your level of obesity, your overall health condition, and your willingness to participate in your weight loss plan. Read on to find out the natural treatment methods that will help you get rid of your extra pounds and live a longer and healthier life.

By: Oliver Greene

Dietary Therapy

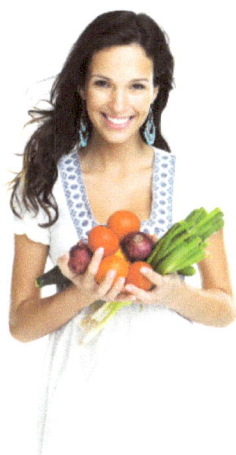

Changing unhealthy dietary patterns, eating healthy food, and reducing calories are vital in order to overcome obesity. It is often due to the discouragement that people quit on eating limited and healthy food. Always remember that weight loss is usually quick at first and tends to become slow and gradual with time. However, reducing one to two pounds per week after cutting down on fatty and sugary food is indeed an achievement and one must not feel discouraged in reducing so less for so much. Reducing weight slowly and gradually over the long term is the most natural and safest way to reduce weight and the best way to keep it off permanently. Avoid unrealistic and drastic changes in diet, such as crash diets, because they are unlikely to keep off excess weight permanently.

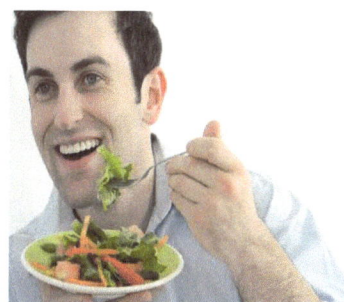

Other dietary ways to prevent obesity include:

Calorie Count – Reducing the amount of calories you consume per day is the key to weight loss. It is wise to assess your eating and drinking habits in order to see the amount of calories you are typically consuming. Assessment will help you determine where you can cut back. You can even seek assistance from your health care provider to help you decide on the right amount of calories that you must consume in order to reduce weight. However, the ideal amount is 1,000 to 1,500 calories per day.

By: Oliver Greene

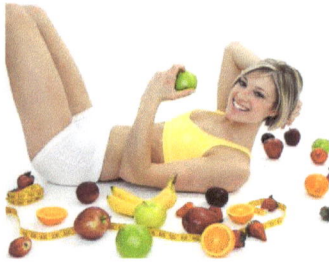

Feeling Full – It is easier to satisfy your hunger without consuming a lot of calories only if you understand the concept of energy density. Every food type has a certain amount of calories. Foods such as fatty and processed foods, candies, and desserts are high in energy density. On the other hand, there are food types, such as vegetables and fruits, which are low in calories. These food items can be consumed in a larger portion without consuming a lot of calories. This means that it is easy to reduce your hunger pangs by eating larger portion of these food items.

Eating Plan – It is very important to choose healthy eating in order to reduce weight. This is possible if you eat more plant-based food, such as vegetables, fruits, and whole grain carbohydrates. Also include sources of protein in your daily diet, such as lean meats, soy and lentils, and beans. Limit added sugar and salt and include fish at least twice a week. If you are consuming dairy products, make sure you consume only low-fat products. While eating fat, keep your quantity to minimum.

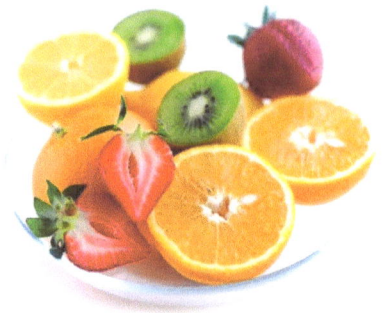

Meal Replacements – There are certain meal replacement products available in the market that suggest to you to replace your meals with their products, such as meal bars or low calorie shakes. Such diets may indeed help you lose weight but these diets likely won't teach your how to implement a change in your lifestyle. Therefore, you will need to keep up with the diet in order to maintain your weight.

By: Oliver Greene

There are many fad diets that guarantee easy and quick weight loss. However, the reality is that there are no such quick fixes or magic food. Fad diets may help in reducing weight on a short term basis, but the long term results don't appear to be very promising.

Similarly, there are crash diets that promise weight loss but you are likely to regain weight as soon as you stop the diet. In order to reduce weight effectively and keep it off permanently, you have to change your lifestyle and adopt healthy eating habits that you can maintain over time.

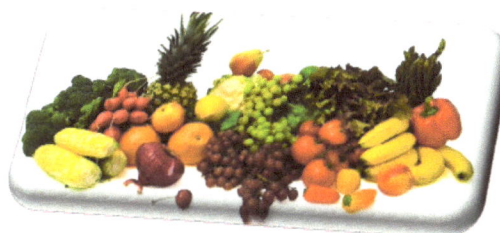

Physical Activity

Increased exercise or physical activity is also an essential part of obesity treatment. People who are able to keep up with their weight loss maintenance for more than a year, usually get used to regular exercise.

To enhance your activity level:

Exercise – According to The American College of Sports Medicine, overweight or obese individuals must at least get 150 minutes of moderate-intensity physical exercise every week in order to lose a modest amount of weight or prevent further weight gain. However, it requires 250 to 300 minutes of high intensity exercise every week in order to achieve significant weight loss. As your fitness and endurance improves, you must also increase the level and duration of your exercise and physical activity. To make your exercise

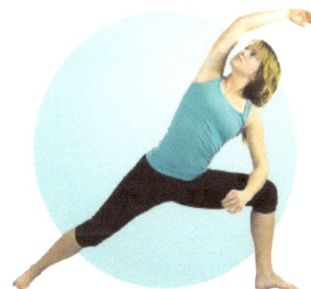

By: Oliver Greene

routine comfortable, break it up into several sessions throughout the day and do only 5 to six minutes at a time.

Daily Activity – Although it is very helpful to indulge yourself into regular aerobic exercise in order to shed excess weight and burn calories, any extra physical activity will also help you achieve weight loss quick. You can earn big benefits by making small and simple changes to your daily routine. Use the staircase instead of the escalator, park farther from the store, look after your garden and household chores, keep track of the steps you take and feel the difference.

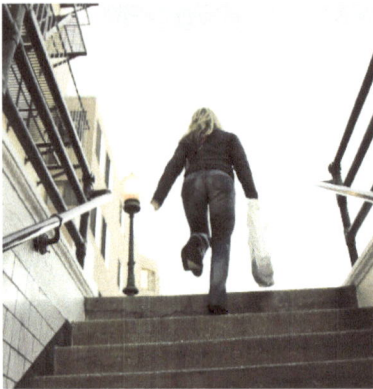

You will only be able to incorporate successful changes in your lifestyle if you are able to see positive results. Therefore, it is very important that you keep a record of your weight for further motivation.

Behavior Therapy

A behavior modification program is vital to bring positive changes to your lifestyle and help you lose weight permanently. Behavior therapy includes assessment of your own habits to find out the situations or factors that are contributing to your obesity.

Behavior therapy or behavior modification includes:

By: Oliver Greene

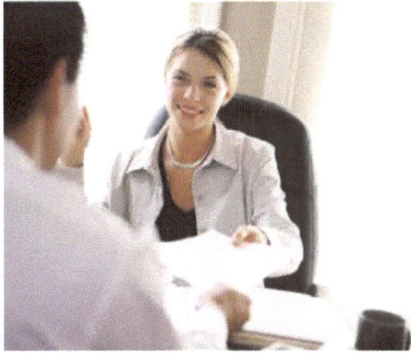

Counseling – Interventions and therapy with medical professionals and mental health professionals can help you address behavioral and emotional issues related to obesity. With therapies you will understand the reasons for your overeating and learn healthy ways to cope with behavioral issues. You can also learn how to cope with food cravings, understand eating triggers, and monitor your activity and diet. Counseling may be available by internet-based programs, email, or telephone if travelling is difficult. Therapy can take place on both group and individual basis.

Support Groups – These groups not only offer you their companionship but also offer you understanding of the similar challenges obese people face. There are many people you will find in these support groups who will share similar problems that you are going through. You can share your ideas, your positive approach towards weight loss and get motivated by others' success stories in the

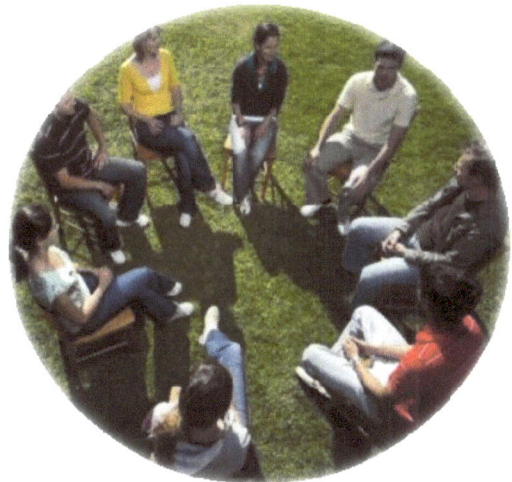

support group. Check with commercial weight loss programs, local hospitals, and your doctor to help you find a relevant support group in your area.

By: Oliver Greene

Support from friends and family contribute a lot to how a person is responding to the lifestyle change. Encourage your friends and family to begin counseling you at home and help you adjust to the changes. Your loved ones can do this by following the same patterns as you are without making it a further challenge for you to give up unhealthy food and following unhealthy lifestyle. Since the changes you are focusing on are positive, it will be healthy for your loved ones to get used to healthy dietary and lifestyle patterns before they even face obesity crisis.

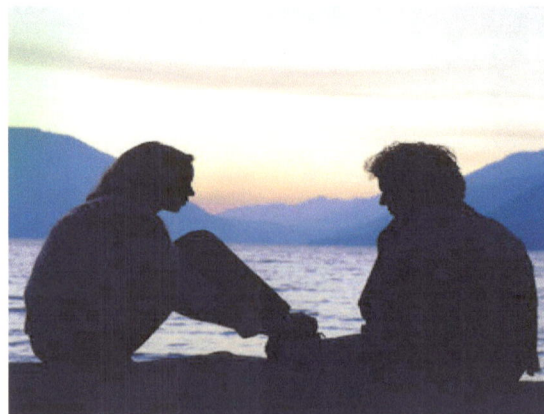

In a nutshell, it is the positive 'approach' that can help you overcome obesity and obesity-related health issues. If you have already decided to change your lifestyle, it is very important to stay determined on the idea. A positive approach together with strong determination will lead you to desirable results.

By: Oliver Greene

Conclusion

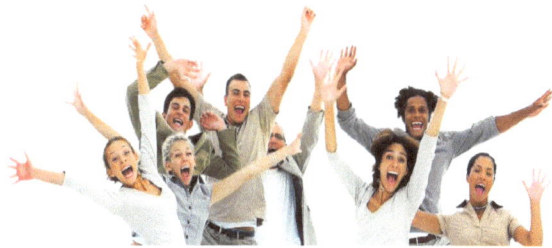

Whether you are overweight, obese, or at your optimum weight, it is very important to learn the causes and health hazards of obesity. Prevention of the causes of obesity is the only way people can fight this growing epidemic and can save their children from becoming victims.

Children who are obese today are increasing the chances of becoming obese adults tomorrow, and obese adults today are encouraging the sedentary lifestyle and unhealthy eating patterns of their children and letting them grow obese. In short, it is a cycle that is allowing obesity to attack our society.

In order to get rid of this growing epidemic, this cycle needs to break. People who are obese today must not only focus on themselves but should also take one step ahead to save their children from following the bad lifestyle that leads to obesity.

People have become couch potatoes and are spending recklessly at fast food chains to satisfy their hunger. Just for a temporary taste on their tongue, people are putting their health and life at stake without even realizing.

This book is a wake-up call to all those slumbering in the deep abyss of obesity. You can still buck up and contribute to saving this planet from the epidemic of obesity.

By: Oliver Greene

We wish you every success in your daily Healthy lifestyle.

Should you require any further help please e-mail me: oliver@the-menace-of-obesity.com

By: Oliver Greene

By: Oliver Greene

www.ingramcontent.com/pod-product-compliance
Lightning Source LLC
Chambersburg PA
CBHW060858270326

41935CB00003B/27